KETO DIET FOR

BEGINNERS OVER 50

40 delicious recipes FOR
WOMEN OVER 50 with a busy
lifestyle who want to lose
weight, improve metabolism
and balance hormones.

By

Samantha Sanchez

Test of Contents

Introduction

Women seeking for a fast and effective way to shed excess weight, get high blood sugar levels under control, reduce overall inflammation, and improve physical and mental energy will do their best by following a ketogenic diet plan. But there are special considerations women must take into account when they are beginning the keto diet.

All women know it is much more difficult for women to lose weight than men to lose weight. A woman will live on a starvation level diet and exercise like a triathlete and only lose five pounds. A man will stop putting dressing on his salad and will lose twenty pounds. It just is not fair. But we have the fact that we are women to blame. Women naturally have more standing between them and weight loss than men do.

The mere fact that we are women is the largest single contributor to why we find it difficult to lose weight. Since our bodies always think they need to be prepared for the possibility of pregnant women will certainly have more body fat and less mass in our muscles than men will. Muscle cells burn more calories than fat cells do. So, because we are women, we will always lose weight more slowly than men will.

Being in menopause will also cause women to add more pounds to their bodies, especially in the lower half. After menopause, a woman's metabolism naturally slows down. Your hormone levels will decrease. These two factors alone will cause weight gain in the post-menopausal woman.

Women are a direct product of their hormones. Men also have hormones but not the ones like we have that regulate every function in our bodies. And the hormones in women will fluctuate around their everyday habits like lack of sleep, poor eating habits, and menstrual cycles. These hormones cause women to crave sweets around the time their periods occur. These cravings will wreck any diet plan. Staying true to the keto plan is challenging because of the intense desire for sweets and carbs. Also, having your period will often make you feel bloated because of the water your body holds onto during this time. And they have cramps make you more likely to reach for a bag of cookies than a plate of steak and salad.

Because we are women, we may experience challenges on the keto diet that men will not face because they are men. One of these challenges is having a weight loss plateau or even experiencing weight gain. It can happen because of the influence of hormones on weight loss in women.

Many women on a keto diet will struggle with imbalances in their hormones. On the keto diet, you do not rely on lowered calories to lose weight but on your hormones' effect. So, when women begin the keto diet any issues, they are already having with their hormones will be brought to attention and may cause the woman to give up before she starts. Always remember that the keto diet is responsible for cleansing the system first so that the body can efficiently respond to the beautiful effects a keto diet has to offer.

Like any other diet plan, the keto diet will work better if you are active. Regular exercise will allow the body to strengthen and tone muscles and help to work off excess fat reserves. But training requires energy to accomplish. If you limit your carb intake too much, you might not have the energy needed to be physically able to make it through the day and still maintain an exercise routine. You might need to add in more carbs to your diet through the practice of carb cycling.

Don't put off getting started. The sooner you begin this diet, the sooner you'll start to notice an improvement in your health and well-being.

The actual act of staying on the keto diet can be very challenging for some women. Many women see beginning a new diet to lose weight as a punishment for being overweight. It may be worthwhile for you to change your mind's settings if you are feeling this way. You may need to remind yourself every day that the keto diet is not a punishment but a blessing for your body. Tell yourself that you do not deny yourself certain foods because you can't eat them, but because you do not like how those foods make your body feel. Don't watch other people eating their high carb diet and pity yourself. Instead, feel sorry for the people who have trapped themselves in a high-calorie diet and are not experiencing the benefits you are experiencing.

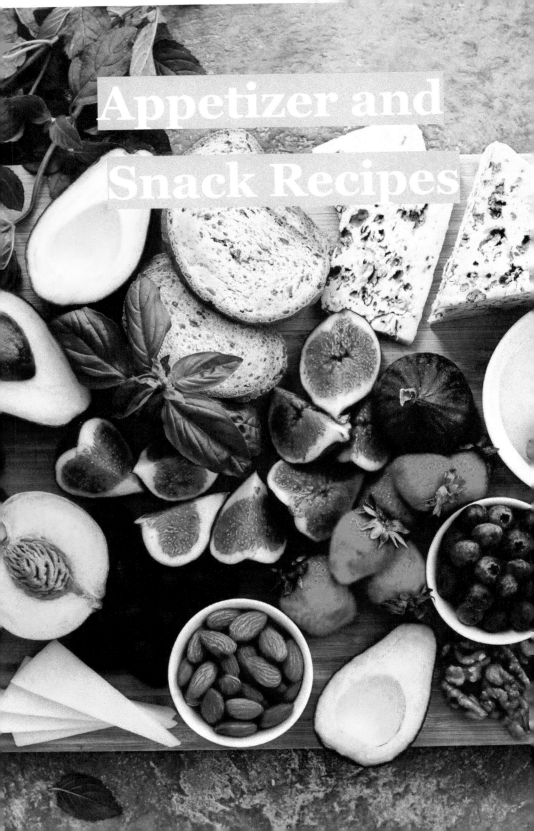

Appetizer and Snack Recipes

1. Delicious Chicken Wings

Preparation Time: 10 minutes

Cooking Time: 30 minutes

Serving: 6

Ingredients:

- 1 egg, beaten

- 1 1/2 lbs. chicken wings

- 6 tbsp olive oil

- 1/2 cup apple cider vinegar

- 1/2 tsp cayenne pepper

- 2 garlic cloves, minced

- 1/2 tsp pepper

- 3/4 tsp salt

Directions:

1. Blend all ingredients except chicken in a large bowl. Add chicken wings in a bowl and mix until well coated and set aside for 20 minutes. Preheat the oven to 450 F.

2. Spray a baking tray with cooking spray. Place marinated wings on a prepared baking tray and bake for 30 minutes. Serve and enjoy.

Nutrition:

355 Calories

23g Fat

0.5g Carbohydrates

2. Lemon Chicken

Preparation Time: 10 minutes

Cooking Time: 45 minutes

Serving: 8

Ingredients:

- 8 chicken breasts, skinless and boneless

- 1/4 cup fresh lemon juice

- 2 tbsp green onion, chopped

- 1 tbsp oregano leaves

- 3 oz feta cheese, crumbled

- 1/4 tsp pepper

Direction:

1. Prepare the oven to 350 F. Spray baking dish with cooking spray. Place chicken breasts in prepared baking dish. Drizzle with 2 tbsp lemon juice and sprinkle with 1/2 tablespoon oregano and pepper.

2. Top with green onion and crumbled cheese. Drizzle with remaining lemon juice and oregano. Bake for 45 minutes. Serve and enjoy.

Nutrition:

245 Calories

10.8g Fat

34g Protein

3. Bacon Appetizers

Preparation Time: 15 minutes

Cooking Time: 1 hour

Servings: 6

Ingredients:

- 1 pack Keto crackers

- ¾ cup Parmesan cheese, grated

- 1 lb. bacon, sliced thinly

Directions:

1. Preheat your oven to 250 degrees F. Arrange the crackers on a baking sheet.

2. Sprinkle cheese on top of each cracker. Wrap each cracker with the bacon. Bake in the oven for 1 hours.

Nutrition:

440 Calories

33.4g Total Fat

29.4g Protein

4. Antipasti Skewers

Preparation Time: 10 minutes

Cooking Time: 0 minute

Servings: 6

Ingredients:

- 6 small mozzarella balls

- 1 tablespoon olive oil

- Salt to taste

- 1/8 teaspoon dried oregano

- 2 roasted yellow peppers, sliced into strips and rolled

- 6 cherry tomatoes

- 6 green olives, pitted

- 6 Kalamata olives, pitted

- 2 artichoke hearts, sliced into wedges

- 6 slices salami, rolled

- 6 leaves fresh basil

Directions:

1. Toss the mozzarella balls in olive oil. Season with salt and oregano. Thread the mozzarella balls and the rest of the ingredients into skewers. Serve in a platter.

Nutrition:

180 Calories

11.8g Total

9.2g Protein

5. Jalapeno Poppers

Preparation Time: 10 minutes

Cooking Time: 75 minutes

Servings: 10

Ingredients:

- 5 fresh jalapenos, sliced and seeded

- 4 oz. package cream cheese

- ¼ lb. bacon, sliced in half

Directions:

1. Ready oven to 275 degrees F. Place a wire rack over your baking sheet. Stuff each jalapeno with cream cheese and wrap in bacon. Secure with a toothpick. Place on the baking sheet.

2. Bake for 1 hour and 15 minutes.

Nutrition:

103 Calories

8.7g Total Fat 8

5.2g Protein

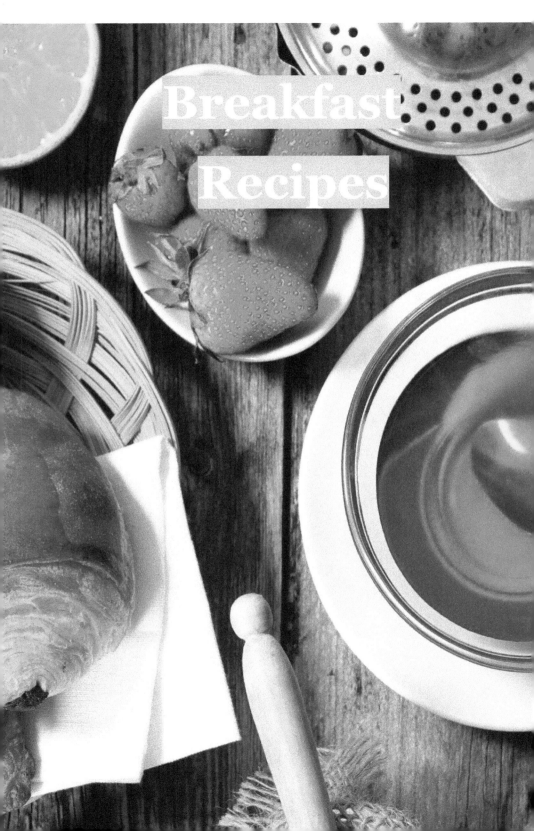

Breakfast

Recipes

6. Bulletproof Chocolate Smoothie

Preparation Time: 3 minutes

Cooking Time: 2 minutes

Servings 2

Ingredients:

- 1 ¼ cup fresh brewed coffee, cooled for at least 15 minutes

- ¼ cup filtered water

- 2 scoops Chocolate Collagen Protein Powder

- 6-8 Ice cubes

Directions:

1. Blend coffee, water and chocolate protein powder until smooth, adding ice cubes until you reach desired consistency.

2. Serve right away.

Nutrition:

30 Calories

1g Fat

7. Basic Bulletproof Coffee Drink

Preparation Time: 2 minutes

Cooking Time: 1 minute

Servings 1

Ingredients:

- 1 cup brewed coffee

- 1 tsp coconut oil

- 1 tbsp butter, unsalted

- ¼ tsp vanilla extract

- A few drops of stevia

Directions:

1. Put all ingredients into blender. Pulse on high for 20 seconds until frothy. Drink immediately.

Nutrition:

148 Calories

14g Fat

8. Strawberry Avocado Green Smoothie

Preparation Time: 5 minutes

Cooking Time: 5 minutes

Servings: 2

Ingredients:

- 1 cup fresh strawberries, hulled

- ½ medium, ripe avocado, peeled

- 1 cup (packed) baby spinach

- 1 cup unsweetened almond milk

- 2 teaspoons sweetener

- 6-8 ice cubes

Direction:

1. Position all ingredients into blender and blend until smooth. Once blended, taste for sweetness and adjust accordingly by adding more strawberries or sweetener as needed. Serve immediately.

Nutrition:

156 Calories

6.9g Fat

2.7g Protein

9. Peanut Butter Cup Smoothie

Preparation Time 5 minutes

Cooking Time: 0 minute

Servings 2

Ingredients:

- 1 cup water

- ¾ cup coconut cream

- 1 scoop chocolate protein powder

- 2 tablespoons natural peanut butter

- 3 ice cubes

Directions:

1. Put the water, coconut cream, protein powder, peanut butter and ice in a blender and blend until smooth. Pour into 2 glasses and serve immediately.

Nutrition:

486 Calories

40g Fat

30g Protein

10.　Green Smoothie

Preparation Time 10 minutes

Cooking Time: 0 minute

Servings: 2

Ingredients:

- 1 cup water

- ½ cup raspberries

- ½ cup shredded kale

- ¾ cup cream cheese

- 1 tablespoon coconut oil

- 1 scoop vanilla protein powder

Directions:

1. Put the water, raspberries, kale, cream cheese, coconut oil and protein powder in a blender and blend until smooth. Pour into 2 glasses and serve immediately.

Nutrition:

436 Calories

36g Fat

28g Protein

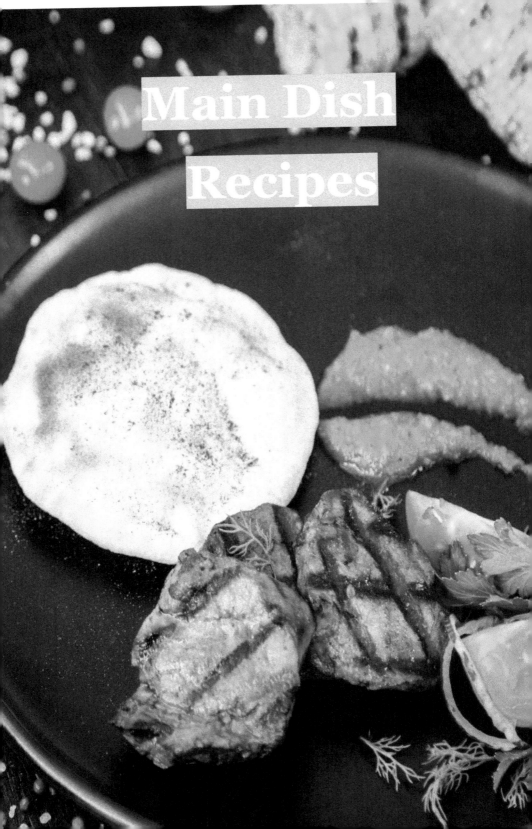

Main Dish

Recipes

11.   Stuffed Chicken Breasts

Preparation Time: 15 minutes

Cooking Time: 30 minutes

Servings: 4

Ingredients

- 1 teaspoon paprika

- ¼ teaspoon onion powder

- ¼ teaspoon garlic powder

- Salt

- 4 grass-fed chicken breasts

- 1 tablespoon olive oil

- 4 ounces cream cheese

- ¼ cup Parmesan cheese

- 2 tablespoons mayonnaise

- 1½ cups fresh spinach

- 1 teaspoon garlic

- ½ teaspoon red pepper flakes

Directions:

1. Preheat the oven to 375°F. Mix spices and salt. Place chicken breasts in cutting board. Drizzle with oil.

2. Rub with spice mixture. Chop pocket into the side of each chicken breast. Mix cream cheese, Parmesan, mayonnaise, spinach, garlic, red pepper, and ½ teaspoon salt.

3. Stuff with spinach mixture. Transfer into a 9x13-inch baking dish. Bake for 30 minutes. Serve.

Nutrition

468 Calories

30.2g Fat

45.7g Protein

12.   Chicken with Capers Sauce

Preparation Time: 15 minutes

Cooking Time: 22 minutes

Servings: 2

Ingredients 2 (5½-ounces) grass-fed boneless

- Salt and black pepper
- 1/3 cup almond flour
- 2 tablespoons Parmesan cheese
- ½ teaspoon garlic powder
- 4 tablespoons olive oil
- 1 tablespoon garlic
- 3 tablespoons capers
- ¼ teaspoon red pepper flakes
- 3–4 tablespoons lemon juice
- 1 cup homemade chicken broth
- 1/3 cup heavy cream

Directions:

1. Season the chicken breasts. Mix flour, parmesan cheese and garlic powder.

2. Cover chicken breasts with the flour mixture. Preheat the oil in wok over medium-high heat and cook for 5 minutes per side.

3. Cover chicken thighs with foil. Pull out oil from the wok, leaving 1 tablespoon inside. Mix capers, garlic, red pepper flakes, lemon juice, and broth.

4. Mix the capers mixture over medium heat. Cook for 10 minutes. Stir in the heavy cream.

5. Return wok over medium heat and cook for 1 minute. Stir in the cooked chicken and remove from the heat. Serve.

Nutrition

783 Calories

59.4g Fat

50.7g Protein

13. Lemony Chicken Thighs

Preparation Time: 10 minutes

Cooking Time: 16 minutes

Servings: 4

Ingredients

- 2 tablespoons olive oil

- 1 tablespoon lemon juice

- 1 tablespoon lemon zest

- 2 teaspoons dried oregano

- 1 teaspoon dried thyme

- Salt and black pepper

- 1½ pounds grass-fed bone-in chicken thighs

Directions:

1. Preheat the oven to 420°F. Mix 1 tablespoon of the oil, lemon juice, lemon zest, dried herbs, salt, and black pepper.

2. Coat chicken thighs with mixture. Marinate for 20 minutes. In oven-proof wok, heat oil over medium-high heat and sear chicken thighs for 3 minutes per side.

3. Situate into the oven and bake for 10 minutes. Serve.

Nutrition

388 Calories

19.7g Fat

49.4g Protein

14.   Bacon-Wrapped Turkey Breast

Preparation Time: 10 minutes

Cooking Time: 1 hour

Servings: 2

Ingredients

- ¾ pound turkey breast

- ½ teaspoons dried rosemary

- ½ teaspoons dried thyme

- ½ teaspoons dried sage

- 6 large bacon slices

Directions:

1. Preheat the oven to 350°F. Ready baking sheet with a parchment paper. Sprinkle with herbs.

2. Wrap the bacon slices around the turkey breast. Place onto the prepared baking sheet and cover with foil.

3. Bake for 50 minutes. Remove the foil and bake 10 minutes. Pull out baking sheet from oven and set aside for 10 minutes.

4. Cut the turkey breast and serve.

Nutrition

345 Calories

6.5g Fat

56.2g Protein

15.   Turkey Meatloaf

Preparation Time: 15 minutes

Cooking Time: 40 minutes

Servings: 8

Ingredients

Meatloaf

- 2 pounds ground turkey

- 1 cup cheddar cheese

- 1 tablespoon dried onion

- 1 teaspoon dried garlic

- 1 teaspoon garlic powder

- 1 teaspoon red chili powder

- 1 teaspoon ground mustard

- 1 organic egg

- 2 ounces sugar-free BBQ sauce

Topping

- 2 ounces sugar-free BBQ sauce

- 5 cooked bacon slices

- ½ cup cheddar cheese

Directions:

1. Preheat the oven to 400°F. Grease 9x13-inch casserole dish.

For meatloaf:

2. Mix all ingredients. Place into the prepared casserole dish and smooth the surface. Coat the top of meatloaf with BBQ sauce evenly and sprinkle with bacon, then cheese.

3. Bake for 40 minutes. Remove from the oven and set aside. Cut the meatloaf and serve.

Nutrition:

380 Calories

21.7g Fat

40.1g Protein

16. Herbed Beef Tenderloin

Preparation Time: 15 minutes

Cooking Time: 30 minutes

Servings: 6

Ingredients

- 4 garlic cloves
- ½ cup fresh parsley
- 1/3 cup fresh oregano
- 2 tablespoons fresh thyme
- 2 tablespoons fresh rosemary
- 2 teaspoons fresh lemon zest
- 6 tablespoons olive oil
- 2 tablespoons fresh lemon juice
- ½ teaspoon red pepper flakes
- Salt and ground black pepper
- 1¾ pounds grass-fed beef tenderloin

Directions:

1. Mix all ingredients except for beef tenderloin. Add the beef tenderloin and coat with the herb mixture. Marinate for 45 minutes.

2. Preheat the oven to 425°F. Remove the beef tenderloin from the bowl and arrange onto a baking sheet. Bake for 30 minutes.

3. Remove the beef tenderloin from oven and place onto a cutting board for 20 minutes. Cut the beef tenderloin and serve.

Nutrition
415 Calories
26.7g Fat
39.2g Protein

17. Steak with Cheese Sauce

Preparation Time: 15 minutes

Cooking Time: 17 minutes

Servings: 3

Ingredients

Steak

- 2 tablespoons fresh oregano

- ½ tablespoon garlic

- 1 tablespoon fresh lemon peel

- ½ teaspoon red pepper flakes

- Salt and ground black pepper

- 1 (1-pound) (1-inch thick) grass-fed boneless beef top sirloin steak

Cheese Sauce

- 2 tablespoons unsalted butter

- 2 garlic cloves

- 1 tablespoon almond flour

- ½ cup homemade beef broth ½ teaspoon dried basil

- ¼ teaspoon dried oregano

- ½ ounce cream cheese

- ¼ cup Parmesan cheese

- ¼ cup heavy cream

- Salt and ground black pepper

Directions:
1. Preheat the gas grill to medium heat. Grease the grill grate. Mix oregano, garlic, lemon peel, red pepper flakes, salt, and black pepper. Rub the steak with garlic mixture.

2. Cook steak onto the grill, covered for 17 minutes.

3. Pull out steak from the grill and set aside for 10 minutes.

For cheese sauce:
4. Sauté butter and garlic in the wok over medium heat. Cook flour for about 1 minute. Stir in broth and dried herbs and cook for about 1 minute.

5. Cook in cream cheese, Parmesan cheese and heavy cream for 1 minute. Season and remove from the heat.

6. Cut the steak into desired sized slices and top with cheese sauce. Serve.

Nutrition

461 Calories

25.9g Fat

50.6g Protein

18.   Steak with Pesto

Preparation Time: 10 minutes

Cooking Time: 10 minutes

Servings: 4

Ingredients

- 1 tablespoon butter

- 4 (6-ounce) grass-fed flank steaks

- Salt and ground black pepper

- ½ cup pesto

Directions:

1. Cook the butter in wok over medium-high heat and cook seasoned steaks for 5 minutes per side.

2. Serve with the topping of pesto.

Nutrition

490 Calories

30g Fat

50.4g Protein

19. Herbed Lamb Chops

Preparation Time: 10 minutes

Cooking Time: 20 minutes

Servings: 4

Ingredients

- 1½ pounds grass-fed lamb loin chops

- 1 tablespoon fresh lemon juice

- ¼ cup fresh parsley

- 2 tablespoons fresh mint leaves

- 1 tablespoon olive oil

- Salt and ground black pepper

Directions:

1. Preheat grill to medium-high heat. Grease the grill grate. Mix lamb loin chops, lemon juice, parsley, mint, oil, salt, and black pepper.

2. Grill for 10 minutes per side. Serve.

Nutrition

350 Calories

16.1g Fat

48g Protein

Side Dish Recipes

20.   Garlic Sautéed Rapini

Preparation Time: 10 minutes

Cooking Time: 11 minutes

Servings: 4

Ingredients:

- 2 tbsp avocado oil

- 4 garlic cloves

- 2 cups (454 g) rapini

For topping

- 1 cup (227 g) grated Monterey Jack cheese

- 2 tbsp toasted almond flakes

Directions:

1. Sauté garlic and avocado oil in a large skillet. Mix in the rapini and cook for 10 minutes. Season with salt.

2. Dish onto serving plates, top with the Monterey Jack cheese, almonds, and serve.

Nutrition:

254 Calories

23.91g Fat

0.6g Fiber

21.   Broccoli Fried Cheese

Preparation Time: 15 minutes

Cooking Time: 14 minutes

Serves: 4

Ingredients:

- 1 (225 g) head broccoli

- 2 eggs

- 1 cup (227 g) grated cheddar cheese

- 1/3 cup (74 g) grated Monterey Jack cheese

- 2 tbsp butter

Directions:

1. Steam broccoli for 10 minutes. Pour the broccoli into a bowl and let cool. Crack on the eggs and mix with the cheeses.

2. Working the batches, melt the butter in a large skillet and fry the broccoli on both sides for 4 minutes per side. Remove the broccoli to a plate and serve warm.

Nutrition:

240 Calories

20.7g Fat

0.3g Fiber

22.   Spicy Butter Baked Asparagus

Preparation Time: 15 minutes

Cooking Time: 15 minutes

Servings: 4

Ingredients:

½ lb. (227 g) asparagus

½ cup (113 g) salted butter

1 tsp cayenne pepper

1 cup grated Monterey Jack cheese

Direction:

1. Ready the oven to 425°F/220°C. Spread the asparagus on a baking tray. Mix the butter, cayenne pepper, salt, and black pepper. Drizzle the mixture on the asparagus and toss well with a spatula. Scatter the Monterey Jack cheese on top.

2. Bake for 15 minutes. Serve afterwards.

Nutrition:

253 Calories

24g Fat

1.3g Fiber

23. Grilled Zucchini with Pecan Gremolata

Preparation Time: 45 minutes

Cooking Time: 8 minutes

Servings: 4

Ingredients:

- 2 zucchinis

- 4 tbsp sugar-free maple syrup

- ½ cup (113 g) olive oil

- 2 scallions

- 8 garlic cloves

- 1 cup (227 g) toasted pecans

- 8 tbsp pork rinds

- 2 tbsp chopped fresh parsley

- 1 tbsp plain vinegar

Directions:

1. Sprinkle the zucchinis with salt and let sit for 30 minutes to release liquid. Pat dry with a paper towel. Mix 2 tablespoons oil with the maple syrup and toss with the zucchinis.

2. Heat a grill pan over medium heat and grill the zucchinis for 4 minutes per side. Put in serving platter.

3. Mix the remaining olive oil, scallions, garlic, pecans, pork rinds, parsley, and vinegar. Spoon the gremolata all over the zucchinis and enjoy!

Nutrition:

852 Calories

84.1g Fat

1.4g Fiber

24. Coconut Cauli Fried Rice

Preparation Time: 10 minutes

Cooking Time: 8 minutes

Servings: 4

Ingredients:

- 2 tbsp coconut oil

- 1 small red bell pepper

- 1 scallion

- 2 garlic cloves

- 4 eggs, beaten

- 1 cup (227 g) cauliflower rice

- 1 tbsp coconut aminos

- 1 cup grated cheddar cheese

Directions:

1. Melt the coconut oil in wok and stir-fry the bell peppers for 5 minutes.

2. Mix in the scallions, garlic and cook for 30 seconds.

3. Scramble eggs to the wok. Mix in the cauliflower rice and cook for 2 minutes.

4. Stir in the coconut aminos, sesame seeds, and adjust the taste. Simmer for 1 minute and stir in the cheddar cheese. Turn the heat off and serve immediately.

Nutrition:

251 Calories

20.68g Fat

1g Fiber

25.   Wild Garlic Skillet Bread

Preparation Time: 50 minutes

Cooking Time: 25 minutes

Servings: 4

Ingredients:

- 3 ¼ cups almond flour

- ¼ tsp erythritol

- ¾ tsp salt

- ¾ oz agar powder

- 1 cup lukewarm water

- 3/8 cup melted butter

- 1 cup chopped fresh wild garlic

Directions:

1. In a mixer's bowl, using the dough hook, mix the almond flour, erythritol, salt, and agar agar powder. Add the lukewarm water and combine until dough forms.

2. Dust a surface with almond flour, add the dough and knead with your hands until smooth and elastic.

3. Brush a bowl with melted butter, sit in the dough and cover with a damp napkin. Put the bowl on top of your refrigerator and let rise for 1 hour.

4. After, take off the napkin and press the dough with your fist to release the air trapped in the dough. Divide the dough into 12 pieces and re-shape into a ball.

5. Grease an oven-proof skillet with olive oil and arrange the dough rolls in the pan. Cover with a damp napkin and rise for 30 minutes.

6. Take off, brush the top of the dough with olive oil, and sprinkle with the wild garlic leaves and some flaky salt.

7. Prep oven to 400°F/200°C.

8. Situate skillet in the oven and bake 25 minutes.

9. Let cool. Enjoy!

Nutrition:

893 Calories

28.6g Fat

0.7g Fiber

26. Crispy Roasted Brussels Sprouts and Walnuts

Preparation Time: 15 minutes

Cooking Time: 14 minutes

Servings: 4

Ingredients:

- 3 tbsp almond oil

- 1/3 lb. (151.3 g) Brussels sprouts

- 2 garlic cloves

- 1 red chili pepper

- 2 sprigs chopped fresh mint

- ¼ cup (59 ml) coconut aminos

- 1 tbsp xylitol

- 1 tbsp plain vinegar

- 1 tbsp toasted sesame seeds

- ½ cup (113 g) chopped toasted walnuts

Directions:

1. Sauté brussels sprouts and sesame oil in a large skillet for 10 minutes.

2. Stir in the garlic, red chili pepper, and mint leaves for 1 minute.

3. Mix the coconut aminos, xylitol, and vinegar. Fill mixture over the vegetables and toss. Simmer for 2 minutes.

4. Mix in the sesame seeds, walnuts, and season.

Nutrition:

351 Calories

37.7g Fat

3.3g Carbs

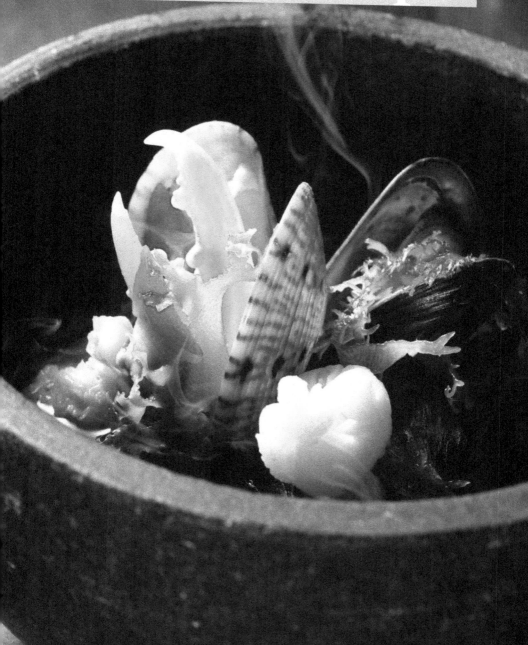

Seafood Recipes

27. Tuna Pickle Boats

Preparation Time: 40 minutes

Cooking Time: 0 minute

Serving: 4

Ingredients

- 1 (5-oz) can tuna, drained

- 2 large dill pickles

- ¼ tsp lemon juice

- 2 tsp mayonnaise

- ¼ tbsp onion flakes

- 1 tsp dill. chopped

Directions

1. Cut the pickles in half lengthwise. Spoon out the seeds to create boats; set aside.

2. Combine the mayonnaise, tuna, onion flakes, and lemon juice in a bowl. Fill each boat with tuna mixture. Sprinkle with dill and place in the fridge for 30 minutes before serving.

Nutrition:

311 calories

12g fat

4g protein

28. Salmon Salad with Lettuce & Avocado (England)

Preparation Time: 5 minutes

Cooking Time: 0 minute

Serving: 3

Ingredients

- 2 slices smoked salmon

- 1 tsp onion flakes

- 3 tbsp mayonnaise

- 1 cup romaine lettuce

- 1 tbsp lime juice

- 1 tbsp extra virgin olive oil

- ½ avocado, sliced

Directions

1. Combine the salmon, mayonnaise, lime juice, olive oil, and salt in a small bowl; mix to combine well.

2. In a salad platter, arrange the shredded lettuce and onion flakes. Spread the salmon mixture over; top with avocado slices and serve.

Nutrition:

112 calories

6g fat

28g protein

29. Mackerel Lettuce Cups

Preparation Time: 10 minutes

Cooking Time: 20 minutes

Serving: 4

Ingredients

- 2 mackerel fillets

- 1 tbsp olive oil

- 2 eggs

- 1 ½ cups water

- 1 tomato, seeded

- 2 tbsp mayonnaise

- ½ head green lettuce

Directions

1. Preheat a grill pan over medium heat. Dash mackerel fillets with olive oil, and sprinkle with salt and black pepper. Add the fish to the preheated grill pan and cook on both sides for 6-8 minutes.

2. Bring the eggs to boil in salted water in a pot over medium heat for 10 minutes. Then, run the eggs in cold

water, peel, and chop into small pieces. Transfer to a salad bowl.

3. Remove the mackerel fillets to the salad bowl. Include the tomatoes and mayonnaise; mix evenly with a spoon. Layer two lettuce leaves each as cups and fill with two tablespoons of egg salad each.

Nutrition:

107 calories

14g fat

27g protein

30. Watercress & Shrimp Salad with Lemon Dressing

Preparation Time: 10 minutes

Cooking Time: 1 hour 10 minutes

Serving: 2

Ingredients

- 1 cup watercress leaves

- 2 tbsp capers

- ½ pound shrimp

- 1 tbsp dill

Dressing:

- ¼ cup mayonnaise

- ½ tsp apple cider vinegar

- ¼ tsp sesame seeds

- 1 tbsp lemon juice

- 2 tsp stevia

Directions

1. Combine the watercress leaves, shrimp, and dill in a large bowl. Whisk together the mayonnaise, vinegar, sesame seeds, black pepper, stevia, and lemon juice in another bowl. Season with salt.

2. Drizzle dressing over and gently toss to combine; refrigerate for 1 hour. Top with capers to serve.

Nutrition:

101 calories

8g fat

21g protein

31. Salad of Prawns and Mixed Lettuce Greens

Preparation Time: 10 minutes

Cooking Time: 15 minutes

Serving: 3

Ingredients

- 2 cups mixed lettuce greens

- ¼ cup aioli

- 1 tbsp olive oil

- ½ pound tiger prawns

- ½ tsp Dijon mustard

- 1 tbsp lemon juice

Directions

1. Season the prawns with salt and chili pepper. Fry in warm olive oil over medium heat for 3 minutes on each side until prawns are pink. Set aside. Add the aioli, lemon juice and mustard in a small bowl. Mix until smooth and creamy.

2. Place the mixed lettuce greens in a bowl and pour half of the dressing on the salad. Toss with 2 spoons until

mixed, and add the remaining dressing. Divide salad among plates and serve with prawns.

Nutrition:

107 calories

4g fat

26g protein

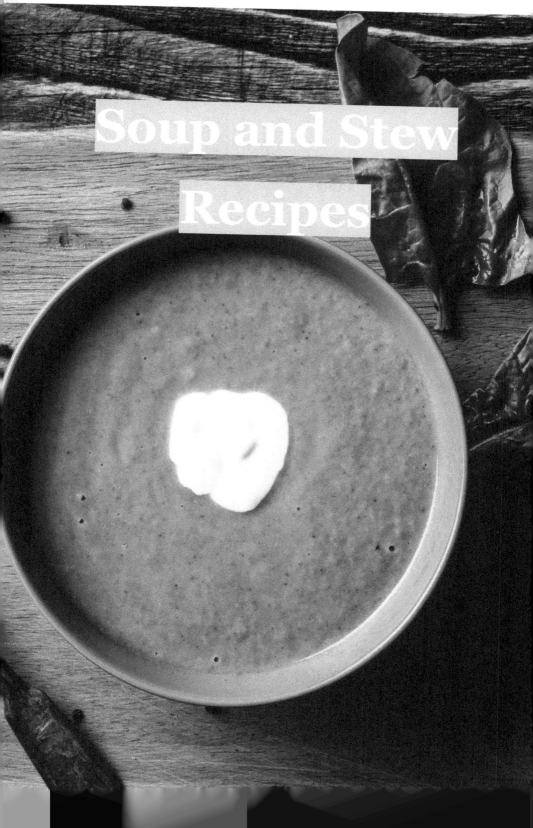

Soup and Stew Recipes

32. Lamb and Herb Bone Broth

Preparation Time: 10 minutes

Cooking Time: 80 minutes

Servings: 8

Ingredients:

- 1-pound lamb bones

- 1 large onion

- 3 medium carrots

- celery stalks

- whole garlic cloves

- fresh sprigs rosemary

- fresh sprigs thyme

- 8 cups of water

Directions:

1. Mix all the ingredients inside your Instant Pot. Lock and cook at high for 50 minutes. When the done, naturally release the tension and remove the cover.

2. Strain the liquid. Transfer the cash to mason jars.

Nutrition:

320 calories

14g fat

38g protein

33. King-Style Roasted Bell Pepper Soup

Preparation Time: 10 minutes

Cooking Time: 25 minutes

Servings: 3

Ingredients

- 4 red bell peppers

- 4 tablespoons olive oil

- 4 garlic cloves

- 1 large red onion

- ¼ cup parmesan cheese

- 2 celery stalks

- 4 cups low-sodium vegetable broth

- 1 teaspoon black pepper

- 1 cup heavy cream

- 1 teaspoon salt

Directions:

1. Preheat your oven to 400 degrees Fahrenheit. Mix the chopped red bell peppers with 2 tablespoons of olive oil.

2. Transfer the red bell peppers to a baking sheet inside your oven.

3. Bake for 10 minutes. Remove from the oven. Set aside. Warmup remaining 2 tablespoons of olive oil over medium-high heat.

4. Sauté the onion, garlic, and celery for 8 minutes.

5. Boil roasted red bell peppers and chicken stock. Close the lid and simmer. Puree the soup. Season it well. Mix in the heavy cream and boil. Remove from the heat. Serve and sprinkle with parmesan cheese.

Nutrition:

317 calories

14g fat

37g protein

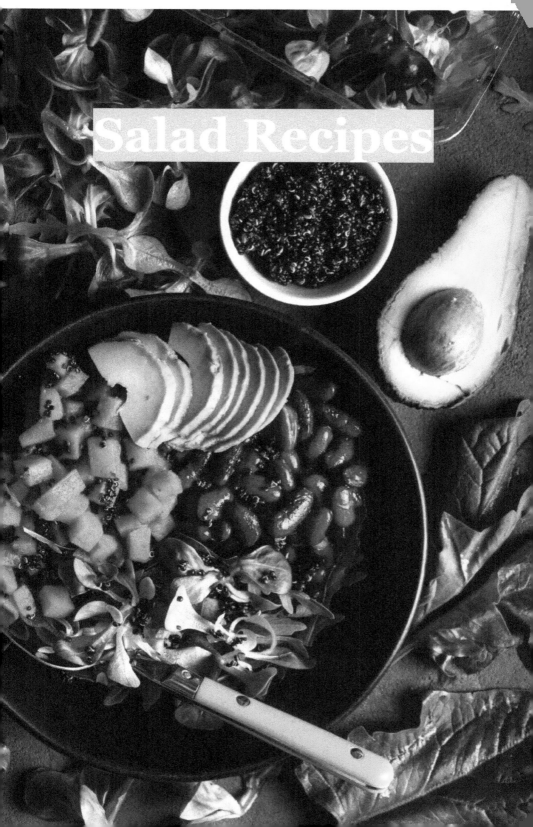

Salad Recipes

34.   Chicken-of-Sea Salad

Preparation Time: 15 minutes

Cooking Time: 5 minutes

Servings: 6

Ingredients:

- 2 (6-oz.) cans olive oil-packed tuna

- 2 (6-oz.) cans water packed tuna

- ¾ C. mayonnaise

- 2 celery stalks

- ¼ of onion

- 1 tbsp. fresh lime juice

- 2 tbsp. mustard

- 6 C. fresh baby arugula

Directions:

1. In a large bowl, add all the ingredients except arugula and gently stir to combine. Divide arugula onto serving plates and top with tuna mixture. Serve immediately.

Nutrition:

325 Calories

27.4g Protein

1.1g Fiber

35.   Yummy Roasted Cauliflower

Preparation Time: 15 minutes

Cooking Time: 20 minutes

Servings: 5

Ingredients:

- 4 C. cauliflower florets

- 4 small garlic cloves, peeled and halved

- 2 tbsp. olive oil

- 1 tbsp. fresh lemon juice

- 1 tsp. dried thyme, crushed

- 1 tsp. dried oregano, crushed

- ½ tsp. red pepper flakes, crushed

Directions:

1. Preheat the oven to 425 degrees F. Generously, grease 2 large baking dishes. In a large bowl, add all the ingredients and toss to coat well.

2. Divide the cauliflower mixture into the prepared baking dishes evenly and spread in a single layer. Roast for about 15-20 minutes or until the desired doneness, tossing 2 times. Remove from the oven and serve hot.

Nutrition:

74 Calories

1.8g Protein

2.3g Fiber

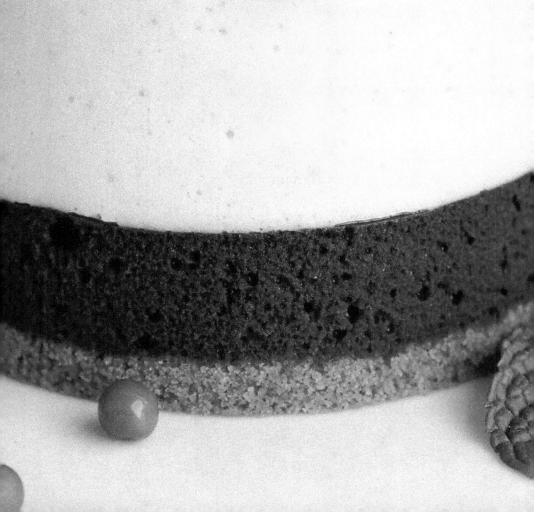

Dessert Recipes

36.   Pumpkin Cheesecake

Preparation Time: 15 minutes

Cooking Time: 80 minutes

Servings: 8

Ingredients:

For Crust:

- 1/2 cup almond flour

- 1 tbsp. swerve

- 1/4 cup butter, melted

- 1 tbsp. flaxseed meal

For Filling: 3 eggs

- 1/2 tsp. ground cinnamon

- 1/2 tsp. vanilla

- 2/3 cup pumpkin puree

- 15.5 oz. cream cheese

- 1/4 tsp. ground nutmeg

- 2/3 cup Swerve

- Pinch of salt Directions:

1. Start to preheat oven to 300 F. Coat 9-inch spring-form pan with cooking spray. Set aside.

For Crust:

2. In a bowl, mix together almond flour, swerve, flaxseed meal, and salt. Add melted butter and mix well to combine. Transfer crust mixture into the prepared pan and press down evenly with a fingertip. Bake for 10-15 minutes. Allow to cool for 10 minutes.

For the cheesecake filling:

3. In a large bowl, beat cream cheese until smooth and creamy. Add eggs, vanilla, swerve, pumpkin puree, nutmeg, cinnamon, and salt and stir until well combined.

4. Pour cheesecake batter into the prepared crust and spread evenly. Bake for 50-55 minutes. Remove cheesecake from oven and set aside to cool completely. Place cheesecake in the fridge for 4 hours. Slices and serve.

Nutrition:

320 Calories

30.4g Total Fat

8.2g Protein

37. Flourless Chocó Cake

Preparation Time: 10 minutes

Cooking Time: 45 minutes

Servings: 8

Ingredients:

- 7 oz. unsweetened dark chocolate, chopped

- ¼ cup Swerve

- 4 eggs, separated

- oz. cream

- oz. butter, cubed

Directions:

1. Grease 8-inch cake pan with butter and set aside. Add butter and chocolate in microwave safe bowl and microwave until melted. Stir well. Add sweetener and cream and mix well.

2. Add egg yolks mix until combined. Beat egg whites in another bowl. Fold egg whites to the chocolate mixture. Bake at 325 F/ 162 C for 45 minutes. Slice and serve.

Nutrition:

318 Calories

28.2g Total Fat

6.6g Protein

38. Gooey Chocolate Cake

Preparation Time: 10 minutes

Cooking Time: 20 minutes

Servings: 8

Ingredients:

- 2 eggs

- 1/4 cup unsweetened cocoa powder

- 1/2 cup almond flour

- 1/2 cup butter, melted

- 1 tsp. vanilla

- 3/4 cup Swerve

- Pinch of salt

Directions:

1. Turn the oven on and preheat to 350 F/ 180C. Spray 8-inch spring-form cake pan with cooking spray. Set aside. In a bowl, sift together almond flour, cocoa powder, and salt. Mix well and set aside.

2. In another bowl, whisk eggs, vanilla extract, and sweetener until creamy. Slowly fold the almond flour

mixture into the egg mixture and stir well to combine. Add melted butter and stir well.

3. Pour cake batter into the prepared pan and bake for 20 minutes. Remove from oven and allow cooling completely. Slice and serve.

Nutrition:

166 Calories

16.5g Total Fat

3.5g Protein

39. Coconut Cake

Preparation Time: 10 minutes

Cooking Time: 20 minutes

Servings: 8

Ingredients:

- 5 eggs, separated

- ½ tsp. baking powder

- ½ tsp. vanilla

- ½ cup butter softened

- ½ cup erythritol

- ¼ cup unsweetened coconut milk

- ½ cup coconut flour

- Pinch of salt

Directions:

1. Start to preheat oven to 400 F/ 200 C. Grease cake pan with butter and set aside. In a bowl, beat sweetener and butter until combined. Add egg yolks, coconut milk, and vanilla and mix well.

2. Add baking powder, coconut flour, and salt and stir well. In another bowl, beat egg whites until stiff peak forms. Gently fold egg whites into the cake mixture.

3. Pour batter in a prepared cake pan and bake in preheated oven for 20 minutes. Slice and serve.

Nutrition:

163 Calories

16.2g Total Fat

3.9g Protein

40. Peach Cake

Preparation Time: 10 minutes

Cooking Time: 20 minutes

Servings: 12

Ingredients:

- 6 eggs

- 2 peaches, stoned, cut into quarters

- 1 tsp. vanilla extract

- 1 tsp. baking powder

- 9 ounces almond meal

- 4 Tbsp. Swerve

- A pinch of salt

- 2 Tbsp. orange zest

- 2 ounces stevia

- 4 ounces cream cheese

- 4 ounces plain Greek yogurt

Directions:

1. Pulse peaches in a food processor. Add Swerve, almond meal, eggs, baking powder, vanilla extract, a pinch of salt, and pulse well. Transfer into 2 spring form pans.

2. Place in an oven at 350F and bake for 20 minutes. In a bowl, mix cream cheese with yogurt, orange zest, stevia, and stir well. Place one cake layer on a plate. Then add half of the cream cheese mixture, add the other cake layer

3. Then top with the rest of the cream cheese mixture. Spread it well. Slice and serve.

Nutrition:

207 Calories

16.5g Fat

8.7g Protein

Conclusion

The utmost goal of the ketogenic diet is to make your body go into a specific metabolic state referred to as ketosis. When body depletes the whole glycogen stores it moves into the fat stores to provide ketones which gives energy to the cells in the body. This means, your body's energy source is no more glucose but the ketones.

But there seems to be a problem here—many people who start with the ketogenic diet have a problem in entering into the ketosis state or staying in the ketosis state after they get in! They often push themselves out of the ketosis state. You can overcome this if you avoid the mistakes that amateurs make.

If you are over 50's, then you know how difficult it is to maintain health and shed that extra weight. Whether you are going through menopause, have more time to eat and socialize, dropping weight after the 50s is not a piece of cake.

If nothing else is working, give the ketogenic diet a try. The fact is that millions of people have successfully implemented a high-fat keto diet as a way to lose weight. It's highly effective because it turns your body into a natural fat burner, without leaving you hungry, craving for sugary foods, or suffering from health effects due to too few calories.

With the keto diet, imagine a life with small belly fat. Imagine eating as much as you want, every single day, and still have small waist and stomach. And, imagine yourself active and energetic as you were in your 20's and 30's.

If you want to lose your extra fat then you will have to take in more fat. Does it sound silly? Well, not if you have heard this — "You have to spend money to make money!"

Keto applies a similar logic—your body needs more dietary fat and extremely fewer dietary carbs to get into ketosis. If you want to change your body to a fat-burning machine, then you should first deprive it of carbs (primary energy source: glycogen—stored glucose). When you do that, your body senses that it has not been getting enough glucose through food and so it starts to use the stored glucose (glycogen). Once it completely exhausts the reserve, it begins to look for an alternate energy source.

Your body targets the stored body fat and breaks it down into fatty acids. These fatty acids produce ketones. When this happens, your body enters into an entirely new metabolic state—ketosis! So, eating more healthy fats is actually going to help you get rid of all the water weight and extra flab. Therefore, you can consume butter and cheese.

If you are a first-time keto dieter, you might experience some of the keto flu symptoms. Constant headaches, fatigue, feeling feverish, etc.—but you do not need to worry, you get these symptoms because your body is trying to adapt to a new routine. It is definitely possible to prevent these flu-like symptoms!

There are few diets that offer you cheat days so that you can wolf down all your favorite stuff on that one day. But beware—there are no cheat days in keto. This is a strict diet routine and you need to adhere to its protocols if you want to achieve your goal weight. If you feel like having a sponge cake or milk chocolate, make a fat bomb and have it.

Keto offers you a substitute for almost everything. Be aware of your mistakes and make preparations accordingly. It is crucial to plan your meals to avoid these commonly repetitive mistakes. Once you get into ketosis, it is not that easy to come out of it but it is not easy to stay on it either!

The important part of any diet is—you should know WHY you are doing it. Are you practicing a particular diet because you want to look good? Or are you doing it to improve your overall health? Whatever the reason is you need to fix it strong in your mind. 99 percent of your diet's success lies in your psychology— your mental capacity should be strong! You need to be sure of why you are doing it and believe that it will work!

CPSIA information can be obtained
at www.ICGtesting.com
Printed in the USA
BVHW050047080421
604338BV00008BA/784

9 781802 450118